T0392266

THE
Divine Dining
Method

21 Days to Transform Your Eating Through
Mindfulness to Create a Happy and Healthy
Relationship with Food . . . for Good

CATHERINE RUSSO EPSTEIN

BALBOA.
PRESS

A DIVISION OF HAY HOUSE

Balboa Press books may be ordered through booksellers or by contacting:

Balboa Press
A Division of Hay House
1663 Liberty Drive
Bloomington, IN 47403
www.balboapress.com
1 (877) 407-4847

Because of the dynamic nature of the Internet, any web addresses or links contained in this book may have changed since publication and may no longer be valid. The views expressed in this work are solely those of the author and do not necessarily reflect the views of the publisher, and the publisher hereby disclaims any responsibility for them.

The author of this book does not dispense medical advice or prescribe the use of any technique as a form of treatment for physical, emotional, or medical problems without the advice of a physician, either directly or indirectly. The intent of the author is only to offer information of a general nature to help you in your quest for emotional and spiritual well-being. In the event you use any of the information in this book for yourself, which is your constitutional right, the author and the publisher assume no responsibility for your actions.

This book is a work of non-fiction. Unless otherwise noted, the author and the publisher make no explicit guarantees as to the accuracy of the information contained in this book and in some cases, names of people and places have been altered to protect their privacy.

Any people depicted in stock imagery provided by Thinkstock are models, and such images are being used for illustrative purposes only. Certain stock imagery © Thinkstock.

Print information available on the last page.

ISBN: 978-1-5043-8763-7 (sc)
ISBN: 978-1-5043-8765-1 (hc)
ISBN: 978-1-5043-8764-4 (e)

Library of Congress Control Number: 2017914270

Balboa Press rev. date: 09/26/2017

To *you*, dear reader, for being a willing participant on your own journey.

To all of you who have crossed my path on this journey of life.

To all my friends, family, and even those who have
challenged me to be the best that I can be!

I'm grateful to all of you who have inspired me to create the most
meaningful programs to help others to live more fully from their hearts.

And to my amazing assistant, Lisa Vetrone, for helping me find order
in my chaotic writings and for keeping me grounded and focused!

Lastly and certainly not least, to my children,
Amanda and Josh, who are my teachers.

Again, to all of you amazing readers, may this book bring you
happiness and *joy*, and may you finally make peace with your food.

CONTENTS

INTRODUCTION
The Divine Dining Method

For over twenty-five years, I've been involved in the self-help and self-growth movements. From humble beginnings in my gem and crystal store to being the founder and CEO of the Living Lotus Group, I'm super passionate about teaching people to make positive choices in their lives, especially when it comes to healthy eating. There is so much more to know about our food struggles and food issues, and each is unique to the individual. There is no magic bullet or simple solution to "fixing" our attitudes toward food.

The Divine Dining Method transcends the traditional approach to eating in that it's not just about what you are eating, but why, how, and when you eat as well. *It is about how you treat yourself while you eat.*

As a transformational life coach who has worked with many people for over twenty-five years, I've developed many different courses and classes to help bring balance back into clients' lives. Since I've struggled with food and weight issues most of my life, I wanted to create products and programs designed to address all the factors that contribute to these eating issues.

My focus is to help people understand their struggles with food and eating issues so that they can develop healthier attitudes toward eating.

Here's a brief history of how the idea of divine dining evolved:

Back in 2006, I developed a workshop called Divine Dining. I taught people how to eat more consciously and mindfully. It was a successful workshop, as many people were new to the term "mindful," especially regarding its relevance to food.

By 2008 I had created the booklet and program to go along with the workshop, and because of my background working with crystal therapy and energy work, I added seven different crystals to serve as reminders of the various aspects of conscious eating. Since that time, I've given countless lectures and helped many people gain control of their eating habits.

If you have ever had the experience of eating something and then realizing you ate the whole bag without tasting it—before proceeding to beat yourself up over it—then *this is the program is for you.*

I too have struggled with making positive and healthy food choices. Many years of fad diets, up and down weight fluctuations, self-help books, gurus, and countless food modification programs had led me to a poor body image and to even poorer self-esteem. One lucky day, though, I read a mindfulness exercise about eating consciously, deliberately, and slowly. Ever the experimenter, I decided to try it myself. I took out an apple, cut it up, and put it on a plate. I carefully chose a slice and examined it before I took the first bite. Then I fully focused on the taste, the crunch, and the chewing (chewing at least twelve times before swallowing). I don't remember how long it took me to eat the apple, but I do remember that it was a pleasant experience. It felt nice to be so tuned in to my food and in control of my eating—but, as life would have it, I moved on with my day and promptly forgot about the *feeling* of that dining experience. Somewhere in the back of my mind, though, the feeling sat and waited patiently to come out again. Soon thereafter, I had a binge session, and in the throes of self-recrimination and judgment, the words *conscious eating* kept repeating themselves. Then one day, while out on a walk (I get my best ideas while out walking or in the shower), the idea of divine dining was born. I wanted to create a comprehensive method to help others nurture a happy and healthy relationship with food. It was also important to teach others how to have healthier attitudes toward eating.

The goals of the Divine Dining Method are to help teach you to:

- ✓ Focus on the food in front of you in the present moment.
- ✓ Pause before the first bite.
- ✓ Be grateful for the food itself.

How to Get the Most Out of This Book

In this book, I will guide you to bringing the divine to the sacred act of eating. Nourish your body with the light of the divine, and see the difference it makes!

Give yourself permission to release your struggle with food and allow more light into your life. Watch what amazing things happen! You will discover that food issues simply cease to exist as you discover that your higher self always guides you to the best choices. Every morsel you put in your mouth becomes a conscious act.

This plan is about creating space and clearing out old energies and programming to make way for the new and amazing *you* that is waiting to shine through. In this plan, the focus is not so much on *what* you eat as it is on *how* you eat. I recommend you choose good quality, organic, and pure foods as often as possible to reap the most benefit from this plan. This not only sets the tone for how you are treating yourself, but it also creates a conscious partnership with those who were responsible for farming, selling, and/or preparing your food.

This is not a diet; it's a supreme act of self-love! I wish you divine dining!

1

What Is the Divine Dining Method?

In the simplest terms, divine dining is a conscious eating program designed to bring your full awareness to the act of eating. It is a program that will help you be aware of what you eat, how you eat, and why you eat.

Have you ever struggled with making healthy food choices? Or are you sometimes unaware of what you are eating until the food is all gone? Do you forget to take the time to enjoy your food? Or do you have food triggers that cause you to go on autopilot or become numb while eating?

If you've answered yes to the above questions and you've been looking to make healthy changes, then the divine dining method is for you!

Divine dining is for you if you have

1) struggled to make healthy food choices;
2) struggled with weight management;
3) eaten on the run, completely unaware of what you're eating until it's all gone;
4) eaten so quickly that you didn't even taste the food;
5) experienced a poor self-image or negative self-talk; or
6) binged or eaten compulsively.

Do You Eat to Live or Live to Eat?

Divine dining helps you identify your food issues and triggers and helps you design the best way to incorporate healthy eating into your life. It helps you be in full control of *what* you eat, *when* you eat, and *why* you eat.

Remember: divine dining is not a diet; it's a supreme act of self-love!

For the purposes of this book, the definition of *mindfulness* is "awareness of the present moment without judgment." Mindfulness is an important part of the Divine Dining Method, as it teaches us to be aware of what we are doing (eating) in the moment.

Q: Why do we want to be more mindful?

A: Because we want to feel we are truly living and not just running through our days on autopilot. We want to be in full control of ourselves and to live more fully from our hearts. We want to be aware of the energy and emotion behind the act of eating. In terms of divine dining, we want to be consistent in the way we approach mealtimes. We want to be aware of what we are eating and why. Knowing ourselves and our motivations for what we are eating is a key to mastering the world of the Divine Dining Method.

2

$\text{\large W}$ho Is It For?

Truthfully, this book is for anyone who eats.

In our society, we are focused on *fast, convenient,* and *easy;* never mind the repercussions these priorities have on our health and well-being. All kinds of people have attended my seminars—thin women, burly men, lifelong yo-yo dieters, and those who don't appear to have a weight problem. I've learned that many issues are related to the act of eating, but not one other approach besides the Divine Dining Method comes even close to mindfulness and conscious eating!

It's important to remember that the Divine Dining Method is a conscious-eating program that is different for everybody. Everyone has different food issues. Some people can't eat when they are stressed; some overeat when they are stressed. Some eat late at night, and some eat while cooking dinner. Once you understand your own issues, you've made the first step in making lasting change.

I'm passionate about helping people understand and accept their food behaviors and getting them to realize that this is the first step in making lasting changes.

I've been inspired by how people have done in our past programs. Here is what a recent client had to say: "The Divine Dining Method taught me to sit and relax while eating and to savor my food instead of rushing through a meal. I was often guilty of leaving the table mid-meal to write a note or put something away. Now I have been treating each meal as a sensory experience."

Here are some of the benefits of adopting the Divine Dining Method:

- ✓ It aids weight loss.
- ✓ It puts you in full control of your eating.
- ✓ It works in conjunction with any eating style.
- ✓ It activates a healthy digestive system.

I have run workshops; held private, individual sessions; and facilitated online virtual retreats, and now, because of my desire to have this program reach more people, I've created an online course that has the entire program in an easy-to-use format. With lessons, a workbook, and meditation recordings, you will have all the support you need to have a successful divine dining experience. You can find the interactive online course at: https://www.lvinglotusgroup.com

You will be inspired in more ways than you could ever imagine in this healing journey, with information and tools to help guide you on your way.

You will come away from this program with many ways to transform your food issues and desires, empowering *you* to make amazing changes. You'll be challenged to confront your existing belief systems and discover how to let go of old patterns while simultaneously opening the way for the new and exciting process of mindful eating to fully take hold in your consciousness.

Here are the top ten reasons for the Divine Dining Method:

- ✓ It's not a diet but a supreme act of self-love. *You get to eat what you want and, more importantly, love what you eat!*
- ✓ It's easy. You don't need special equipment (the crystals are an added bonus but not necessary), scales, weigh-ins, or food portions.

✓ It's portable. Take your mind with you, and you'll be present no matter where you are. As Jon Kabat Zinn said, "Wherever you go, there you are."

✓ It teaches compassion and self-acceptance. What's not to love?

✓ The Divine Dining Method lasts your entire lifetime.

✓ It teaches being nonjudgmental—a helpful technique that will serve you well.

✓ It really works! I love speaking to people after they've been doing the DD Method for a while. It changes your brain in relation to how you approach mealtimes.

✓ It helps create balance. When you are mindful in one area of your life, you are more aware in other parts of your life. It helps to bring balance to your mind, body, and emotions.

✓ Anyone can do it!

✓ It's a positive approach, focusing on how to eat rather than on what not to eat. This is an important distinction and one that helps shift your mind-set and train your brain in a gentle way.

3

*W*hat Are the Benefits?

The Divine Dining Method is a conscious way to transform your mealtime. By working with mindfulness, meditation, affirmations, and crystals to use as energetic touchstones or reminders, you will be guided to be more conscious and aware of your eating.

Here's a note by a recent Divine Dining Method participant: "The Divine Dining [Method] has brought much awareness to an area of my life wrought with old patterning, addiction, and unconscious behavior. Your program has allowed me to gently, compassionately shift my behaviors to ones that are more supportive and uplifting to my entire being. I try to practice once a day, and there are days when there is no consciousness at all to my eating, but my self-awareness is growing along with my self-care and self-love."

We all need to eat, right? If you've had issues with food (and who hasn't?), you might find the following list of benefits to be helpful.

The amazing benefits of the Divine Dining Method include the following:

- ✓ The Divine Dining Method aids in weight management.
- ✓ The Divine Dining Method is not a diet but a supreme act of self-love that teaches us to be kinder to ourselves.

- ✓ The Divine Dining Method works in conjunction with any eating style.
- ✓ The Divine Dining Method is about the intention that we put behind the act of eating.
- ✓ The Divine Dining Method activates a healthy digestive system.
- ✓ The Divine Dining Method reminds us that chewing completely and thoroughly before swallowing will help to stir the digestive juices.
- ✓ The Divine Dining Method encourages us to be in full control of *what* we eat (making healthy choices), *when* we eat (noting time of day, etc.), and *why* we eat (watching for emotional eating).

Why I Created This Program

Our deepest self-knowledge resides in the body, which a great deal of the time does not speak the same language as the mind.

—Annemarie Colbin,
founder of the National Gourmet Institute

How often do you listen to your body? Do you consistently make food choices that are not aligned with your intentions of living a healthier lifestyle?

I am the founder of the Living Lotus Group, a dynamic resource for transformational tools of spiritual growth. A New York-based company rooted in holistic healing and mindful living, Living Lotus Group provides classes, workshops, and meditations; one-on-one and group services, such as life-coaching, reiki, and sound healing; and artisanal jewelry, healing stones, crystal kits, and more through its retail branch, Jewels of the Lotus. As a transformational life coach who helps people align with the lives they want, I have studied various forms and modalities of personal development. One of the recurring themes among my clients has been not living in alignment with their thinking and behavior. People who say they want to eat more healthy foods behave in ways that run counter to their desired outcomes.

I created the Divine Dining Method in 2006 and began teaching workshops to help people who struggle with food issues learn conscious, mindful ways to eat so that they can learn to have healthier attitudes toward eating.

If I were to simplify the Divine Dining Method, I would tell you to try these three tips:

✓ *Focus* on the food you eat while you are eating.
✓ *Pause* and take a deep breath before your first bite.
✓ *Appreciate* and be *grateful* for your food (where it came from and who prepared it).

Ten Ways That the Divine Dining Method Can Change Your Life

Here are some of the many benefits that will influence your body, mind, and soul! The Divine Dining Method supports your efforts to slow down in a busy world and reconnect with your heart center.

✓ The Divine Dining Method teaches you to be more mindful of the wonderful and healthy food with which you choose to nourish your body.
✓ The Divine Dining Method activates a healthier and more balanced digestive process.
✓ The Divine Dining Method helps bring conscious awareness to the energy you put into the act of eating and encourages you to eat your food with *love* and *gratitude*.
✓ The Divine Dining Method transforms the way you view food and how you choose to eat.
✓ The Divine Dining Method assists you in honoring mealtime as a special and sacred event (even if you dine alone).
✓ The Divine Dining Method encourages you to be in full control of your eating (and thereby limits overeating).
✓ The Divine Dining Method increases your awareness of the full range of your emotions and other triggers.

- ✓ The Divine Dining Method deepens your conscious connection to where your food was sourced from and how it was prepared.
- ✓ The Divine Dining Method aligns you with the wisdom of your body, helps you enjoy the foods you love, and teaches self-compassion.

4

$\mathcal{M}$ind-Set and Preparations

Getting Started

Now is the time to sweep away all your feelings of failure and your past perceived mistakes. The joy of the Divine Dining Method is that we get to begin anew in each moment.

The best way to start is to begin with acceptance. By accepting yourself completely, you acknowledge that you are the total sum of all your past successes, lessons, trials, and experiences, but you don't let that story define you.

Mind-Set: The Five Quickest Ways to Shift Your Relationship with Food

When you think about it, we all need to eat to stay alive and stay healthy. Sometimes our intentions don't quite match up with our desires, which is where the problems lie. Let me explain: Our intention is to have healthy bodies, yet we eat foods that are not healthy for us. While the reasons behind this can run deep, it all comes down to following a few simple steps.

1) Be aware of your self-talk when you eat. Do you feel guilty or sneaky, or do you enjoy every bite? This is key to making a shift. Awareness and gentleness come first.

2) Be grateful for your food. Appreciate where it came from. Take a pause before you take the first bite. Learn to slow down.

3) Be conscious of your body while you eat. Learn to check in with your body and stop eating when you are full.

4) Be focused fully on the food in front of you. Try to absorb the smell, the taste, and the texture.

5) Be patient with yourself. Learn to choose healthier options and to enjoy what *life* tastes like.

Seven Skills of Divine Dining (Mindful Eating)

This section is adapted from *Eat, Drink, and Be Mindful* by Susan Albers. The seven skills of mindful eating include the following:

1) Awareness. Awareness is the key to this process. It means we are fully awake and engaged in our eating from start to finish. It means that even if we are choosing to eat something we know is a trigger, at least we are aware of it. (Compare this to the times you've eaten yourself into a stupor and didn't realize it until the bag of chips was empty.) I find that awareness is an important first step because it means that we can make fully informed choices. We are aware of our triggers, old patterns, familial tendencies, and emotional landscapes.

2) Observation. The skill of observation teaches us to separate ourselves from the activity. Almost as if watching ourselves from above, we get to observe (again, without judgment) our tendencies and even what is going through our minds at any given moment. Observe how you speak to yourself, convince yourself, or even lie to yourself! This can be an informative skill.

3) Presence. Our minds can take us on such wild rides during the day, but developing the skills of mindfulness helps bring our full presence into the day. One example is driving. When we are first learning to drive, we are more focused on all the components going into driving (and on wanting to do it right so as not to crash the car). Once we get more experience, we do

it on autopilot. Sometimes we arrive at our destinations without remembering how we got there! When we eat, it's important to be in the moment—not thinking about the past or the future but keeping the focus on the *now*. Multitasking is not being in the present moment. Your attention is split, so it's hard to maintain full focus. Ultimately, presence means being fully focused on what you are eating—not on watching television or reading the paper. Full engagement in the act of consuming your food is a goal to strive for.

4) Being mindful of the environment. Do you eat in your car? (I've done it many times.) Is your dining room table a catchall for the mail and homework gremlins? Creating a nice and peaceful environment for your meals is an important aspect of the Divine Dining Method. Setting the table and creating an atmosphere of love and respect for yourself and your dinner companions will enhance the experience. Do you keep healthy foods in your pantry, or are you being tempted into sabotage?

5) Being nonjudgmental. "Be kind to yourself!" When I say this to clients, they look at me with surprise as if they had just been caught red-handed. I'm big on calling people out on their behaviors, and it's amazing to me how poorly some people treat themselves. This kind of negative self-talk is usually based on early imprinting and carries over into adulthood. Catch yourself when you hear this critical voice come up that says, "I've never been good at ..." Learn how to reframe it into a positive statement, such as, "I love learning a new way to be." It's time to take the boxing gloves off. Start treating yourself with compassion.

6) Letting it go. It's time to stop labeling things as "good" or "bad" and to start recognizing the impermanence of all things—including strong feelings. When we learn how to recognize the pull of a craving or of a food trigger, we can learn other ways of coping with these seemingly overwhelming feelings. For me, one way of "letting go" is to fully immerse myself so that I can *feel the feeling*, as intense as it may be. Instead of wanting to eat my way through it, deny it, or numb it out, I simply breathe through it and let it pass through me. Detach and let go. This is not always

easy when we are in the throes of our emotions, but it is part of our practice.

7) Acceptance. We humans are never truly satisfied with what we have. Many people have something they'd like to change about themselves. Given the choice, they'd wish to be taller or shorter or have better hair or even have more hair. Many people wish their noses weren't so big or that if they could just "lose those last 10 pounds," they'd be happy. In reality, part of compassion is fully accepting ourselves as we are—warts and all! Start with accepting yourself in all your glory! You really are a special human being with unique gifts. It's time to have the courage and the conviction to move in the direction of self-compassion and self-respect. It's time.

As you begin to embark on the Divine Dining Method, you can make space for a new and higher way to approach eating.

5

The Divine Dining Method Seven-Day Conscious Eating Plan

Divine Dining (Mindful Eating)

Conscious eating is about the relationship you have with yourself and your relationship with food. It is the art of bringing your full attention to the act of eating.

Imagine you are in full control of *what* you eat, *when* you eat, and *how* you eat. Visualize that you are fully present in the process of eating and are thoroughly enjoying the act of eating. Conscious eating teaches us to be mindful of the tastes, aromas, and sensations of food and thus becomes a meditation. When you engage all your senses, you can bring about positive changes in your approach to food and become healthier in all areas of your life. Food is what sustains us and energizes us; it fills our souls as well as our bellies. When we bring the *intention* of making mealtime a sacred experience, our connection to the inner self is enhanced.

When you instill a conscious eating habit in your life, you'll be kinder to your digestive system, and you won't overeat. You'll be in tune with your body and will learn to stop when you are full. If you aren't ready to make a whole transformation of your eating habits, then try it with a snack or a light meal. Food can become a spiritual experience when it is approached from a mindful perspective.

Make your mealtime a blessed event. Sit down, even when you are eating by yourself. Before you begin to take the first bite, breathe deeply. Give thanks for your life, your body, and your lessons. Pick up the utensil with reverence, and inhale the aromas deeply. As you begin to eat, make sure you chew thoroughly and taste all the flavors. Imagine the love and the nourishment fulfilling you as you keep chewing. To aid digestion, it is suggested that you chew each bite between twelve and thirty times.

Be mindful of the food in front of you; approach meals with a grateful heart, and you will bring your eating under control. Remember, even if you practice mindfulness at just one meal, it is a start. Release your struggles, allow them to be transmuted by the universal divine light, and remember to honor yourself and your body!

The Divine Dining Method Seven-Day Conscious Eating Plan

This workbook is easy to use. Each day has a specific corresponding crystal for the morning meditation (take at least five to ten minutes for this meditation). The suggested crystals have specific energetic properties that will help serve as a reminder for you to adhere to the Divine Dining Method.

There is space at the end of each page to record your meals, thoughts, insights, and musings.

Before you begin, here are some points to remember:

- ✓ This is a gift you are giving yourself.
- ✓ It is not necessary to weigh in.
- ✓ Open your heart to gratitude and bless your food.
- ✓ Before eating, ask yourself if you are truly hungry.
- ✓ Make mealtime a sacred time, and be sure you are sitting down. (Leaning over the sink doesn't count!)

✓ Remember to take full, deep breaths before, during, and after each meal.

✓ Chew every bite thoroughly (twelve to thirty times to begin the digestive process—or as much as you can) and *swallow* before going on to the next bite.

✓ Engage the senses: make sure the food smells good and is visually appealing; fully enjoy its texture and of course, taste. (You can hear the sound of food as you chew it.)

✓ If you are preparing your food, bring your full awareness to the act, and be mindful during the cooking process.

✓ Be compassionate with yourself; if you get off track, start again at the next meal. This is about doing things differently. (We get a fresh start in each moment!)

✓ Use the suggested affirmations or come up with your own!

Meditation

Do this daily for five to ten minutes.

✓ Relax the body and allow the breath to take you deep within.

✓ Ask your angels and guides to surround you with loving protection.

✓ Bring your attention into your center and see your inner light.

✓ Imagine that your food addictions, struggles, and negative habits are in front of you.

✓ See them being released and dissolved by the divine light.

✓ Ask your higher self to be with you and help you with this transition as you make your way toward healthier eating.

✓ Imagine that you see yourself before you begin to eat. See yourself pausing before you begin to put the food into your mouth.

✓ Know you can make positive food choices that are loving to yourself.

✓ Feel the energy within, and let it fill you.

✓ Continue to take deeper breaths for a few moments.

✓ Know that you are always supported and loved by the divine.

Day One: Clear Quartz Crystal

This is the day you set your intention and clarify your plan to the universe. You are no longer going to struggle with choosing the right foods. You are going to allow yourself to have the freedom to eat whatever you select. The only thing you must remember is to focus on the act of eating. *Completely.*

Clear quartz helps bring clarity to the mind and helps release blockages. Holding your quartz, begin with deep breathing. As you get centered and feel yourself becoming focused, actively set your intention to approach food with a new attitude. This is the first step toward freedom, and it is powerful. Breathe in, and feel fully aligned with this intention. Choose whatever words are appropriate and comfortable to you.

Today's Affirmation

"My eating habits are healthy and nurturing."

Day Two: Rose Quartz

Set the intention to flood your body with self-love and to break the old patterns and conditioning. Your only goal on this day is to bring love into the act of eating. When you focus on this act, your awareness fully illuminates all the senses. Open your heart center and see the divine love emanating from there. Let it envelope you and surround you. Breathe it in.

Hold your rose quartz, and sense a gentle pulsation in your hand. Gently see and feel this pulsating energy rising up your arms and enveloping you in pure love.

Today's Affirmation

"I am filled with the light and love of the divine."

Day Three: Yellow Calcite

Today is the day you align your will with divine will, which can help remind you to stay the course. Yellow calcite helps the solar plexus (which is the third chakra, our sense of self) to open. It allows us to be who we are in a healthy way and is supportive of the supreme nurturing of ourselves. When we are comfortable with ourselves and act from a place of love instead of fear, we bring about great changes in our lives. Yellow calcite also reminds us to bring in more joy!

Today's Affirmation

"I am in alignment with my higher purpose."

Day Four: Carnelian

This stone helps balance the emotional center, or the second chakra, where we process so much of the world around us. This is the center where addictive patterns lie; by letting go of these old patterns, we create space for new and healthy ones to come into our lives. Carnelian helps to bring these positive changes!

Today's Affirmation:

"I consciously choose new and nurturing ways to nourish my body."

Day Five: Aventurine

Celebrate how far you have come, and allow yourself to feel your growth. Aventurine has a soothing and calming energy to help allow your heart to fill with the joy and beauty within. This stone has a soft energy that will help you integrate the work you have done so far. There is joy in the inner depths of your soul! Let that feeling dance in and around you.

Today's Affirmation

"I celebrate my growth and allow what is best for me."

Day Six: Selenite

Selenite helps you link with your higher self to continue to tune into your body and its needs. Remember to breathe in the pure white light of the divine. This is the energy that will nourish and sustain you. Selenite can open the connection to inner wisdom and spur you to live more fully as your true, authentic self. The more light we bring into our lives, the more we can evolve spiritually.

Today's Affirmation

"I am living as my true, authentic self."

Day Seven: Hematite

Get ready to shine your inner light and inner beauty out to the world. Be authentic in who you truly are and allow that to reflect back at you. This plan has been about creating space and clearing out old energies and programming to make way for the new and amazing *you* who is waiting to shine through.

Use the hematite to reflect back your beauty.

Today's Affirmation

"The light of the divine shines within me."

Food for Thought

"The journey of food begins long before it appears sanitized, frozen, processed, prepared and packaged neatly on your grocery shelves. Food all begins alive, in the world, swimming in rivers and oceans, grazing on ranches, growing on trees, and ripening in fields. Too often we think of food just as any manufactured product, when in truth it is of the earth, like all of us. If you really think about it, the wholeness of food is dependent on an entire community that is responsible for getting food on our table.

Then there are those who distribute and ship the food to our local communities. The effort is massive and seamless, which is why it is easy for us- unlike countries less fortunate- to take our bounty for granted."

—Donald Altman, *Meal by Meal*

Food for Thought

"Let's say you are going to eat some chocolates. It's likely that one isn't enough. You won't feel really satisfied. But eating ten of them, as you may have found out in the past, is way too many. Eating this many has previously led you to feel sick; you can have too much of a good thing! So, the next time you eat too many chocolates (or whatever food you are eating), use this information as a starting point. Try to reduce the number by even just one or two, If ten were too many, are seven "just enough"? Is this a satisfying amount? Continue to practice until you find the comfortable amount."

—Susan Albers, "Mindful Eating Tip: Find Your Satisfaction Zone," *Eat, Drink, and Be Mindful*

As you begin to embark on using the Divine Dining Method, you can make space for a new and higher way to approach your eating.

Food for Thought

"Do you identify more strongly with your physical body or your "energy" body? Each approach affects how you eat and the emotions you feel around eating. If you worry a lot about how your body looks, fret over dress or pants size, and always think about how much (or little) you eat, then you identify with the physical body. Do you see how this approach is outward-focused? In addition, it is difficult to hold the physical body up to an ideal because it is always changing and aging. But it you experience yourself as energy, then you will be concerned with getting enough aerobic exercise and eating food that nourishes you with uplifting energy. Food's purpose shifts to the longevity and health of your energy body. This is because the energy body manifest and maintains the physical body. So while good energy food will help your physical body- only you can let go some of the worry."

—Donald Altman, *Eating for Your Energy Body: Meal by Meal*

How well do you know your eating style? Do you worry while you eat?

Food for Thought

"The first thing to do when you sit down with your bowl of food is to stop the thinking and be aware of your breathing. Breathe in such a way that you are nourished. You are nourished by your breathing and you nourish other people with your breathing. We nourish one another."

—Thich Nhat Hanh, "Breathing Comes First," *How to Eat*

How often do you notice your breath while you eat? Is it shallow, deep, or somewhere in between?

6

Secrets to the Divine Dining Method

The following steps are all you'll need to be successful in the Divine Dining Method. Read each one slowly and carefully. Commit them to memory. Until you do, print this out and keep this reminder with you.

Remember: P R A Y E R

P—*pause* before you take the first bite.
R—*reflect* on the food in front of you.
A—*appreciate* the food and its source.
Y—*you* (remember *you* are divine).
E—*eat* with intention, and en*joy* your food.
R—*remember* to breathe.

Recipe for Successful Divine Dining

To successfully engage in the Divine Dining method, use the following recipe:

Start with a healthy cup of acceptance for who you are.

Catherine Russo Epstein

Add a sprinkling of compassion.

Toss in some nonjudgmental, healthy attitudes, and notice any self-sabotage.

Combine with some breath awareness mixed with a full measure of focused, mindful attention to your food.

Enjoy! Focus on the TASTE, an acronym that stands for the following: temperature, aroma, seed at which you eat, texture, and the energy you put into eating (are you eating out of guilt?).

7

Frequently Asked Questions and Crystal Properties

FAQs

Q: I rarely eat lunch at home, what should I do?

A: Take the daily card and the crystal with you as a reminder.

Q: Is it okay to read while you eat?

A: The program works best if you give your full attention to the act of eating, as this allows your focus to be on one thing at a time. This is hard for most people, so try it at one meal to start.

Q: I've finished the seven-day cycle and loved it; now what?

A: You can either do the program again from the beginning or choose a stone with the corresponding affirmation that you love. It is best to keep it going until it becomes ingrained into your life.

Q: Can I do this with a specific diet?

A: Absolutely! If you are trying to lose weight, this is a wonderful way to incorporate mindfulness with a specific food program. That way you combine the physical, emotional, and spiritual aspects of eating.

Q: I haven't been able to follow this method at every meal; should I continue?

A: This plan is a significant change to the way most people approach meals, so please allow room for adjustment. Every moment is a chance to start fresh, so be gentle with yourself. Even if you can only be mindful at one meal, you are taking a step toward a more conscious life!

Q: Sometimes I feel guilty that I've eaten something I shouldn't have; what do I do with that feeling?

A: Remember that your intention is the most important concept and that the energy you put into the act of eating is key. Instead of feeling guilty about your choice, shift into fully enjoying that piece of chocolate (or whatever) and bring all your awareness into play. When you do this, it changes the experience! In other words, if you are going to eat it, make a choice to be fully present.

Crystal Properties

Clear Quartz

Clear quartz brings clarity to the mind and helps us set intentions. It also helps remove blockages.

Rose Quartz

Rose quartz is a gentle yet powerful heart-healing stone. It allows us to open our hearts to receive more love, and it helps surround us with loving energy.

Yellow Calcite

Yellow calcite is a stone that allows us to open to joy. When we are aligned with the divine will, we are in flow with all that is for our highest and best good. Calcite helps release blockages in the solar plexus so that more of our true divine selves can shine!

Carnelian

Carnelian works on an emotional level and helps clear out any blockages. It also helps strengthen the second chakra and release any old patterns or addictions.

Aventurine

Another heart-healing stone, aventurine works gently with the emotions. It soothes and calms, and it can serve to remind us of how far we have come.

Selenite

Selenite is a stone that helps us integrate our higher selves into the physical plane. Using this stone helps bring in the pure white divine light. It is a stone that can scratch easily. Also use care not to let it get wet, as it will dissolve.

Hematite

Hematite is a grounding and protective stone that is great for circulation issues. It helps us remember that words and actions affect everyone around us, and it reminds us of our divinity. Hematite helps us shine our inner light brightly!

8

What's Next?
The Seven-Day Method
Journal and Workbook

Isn't it amazing how far you've come in just the first seven days? Once you are awake and aware, it becomes more difficult to fall back into old, sleepy ways. If you do, that small and nagging voice will continue to make you feel uncomfortable until you heed the call to get back on track.

Welcome to the Divine Dining Method Workbook!

This is the exercise guide to the Divine Dining Method Seven-Day Conscious Eating Plan and is meant to accompany the entire kit. Used as an adjunct to the rest of the book, this workbook gives you seven additional questions to delve deeper into your emotional issues and triggers. Utilize this workbook to take notes and to jot down your personal experiences. Each day has a journal prompt or a question to get you to think about your eating habits and triggers. Feel free to write in the space provided, or choose your own special journal for this program.

Before you begin, here are some key points to remember:

- ✓ Mindfulness is full awareness of the present moment without judgment.
- ✓ Become aware of your beliefs about food and eating, and contemplate where they came from.
- ✓ You are likely learning a whole new way of eating, so be gentle with yourself.
- ✓ Stay focused on your breath.
- ✓ Bless your food before you begin to eat.
- ✓ Journaling thoughts, feelings, and emotions can help you stay on task. (Find a safe and quiet place to let your writing flow.)
- ✓ Honor your hunger.
- ✓ Be *grateful* for your food.

****

Four Foundations of Mindful Eating

Ponder these foundations as you integrate them into your eating rituals.

Mindfulness of the Mind

Nurturing mindfulness of the mind means being aware in any given moment and observing the tastes, smells, and texture as you eat.

Mindfulness of the Body

Nurturing mindfulness of the body means paying attention to what your body is telling you and observing how you are feeling. Do you stop eating when you are full?

Mindfulness of Feelings

Nurturing mindfulness of feelings means noticing if any feelings trigger you before you eat. Are you feeling anxious or bored? Stressed out or angry?

Mindfulness of Thoughts

Nurturing mindfulness of thoughts means asking yourself questions, such as the following: What do you think about while you eat? Are your thoughts compassionate, nonjudgmental, or critical?

> *Your worst enemy cannot harm you as much as your own unguarded thoughts.*
>
> —Buddhist saying

This workbook is an appendix to the seven-day eating program, as it helps you dive deeper into identifying your eating issues. The following journal prompts and exercises will help inspire you and stimulate your thinking. There is plenty of space for you to journal your reflections; also feel free to grab a journal or blank pages to add if you wish.

Daily Check-in Exercise: Get Out of Your Head and into Your Heart

Stop for a moment, and close your eyes. Do an inner check-in in which you ask these questions in order:

1) What am I feeling?
2) What do I want or need?
3) What's my next step?

Bypass the thinking mind, and let your first answer come up. It is always an interesting surprise when we open ourselves to hear ourselves! Journal what comes up for you each time you do this. Write your reflections here:

Day One: Begin with Intention

Write down your intention for this journey. Think about what you want to achieve and how you will feel after you gain control of your eating habits. Use an index card or a sticky note that you are sure to see at least three times a day. Speak your intentions out loud, as that will help further impart them to your consciousness. Each intention could be as long or as short as you wish. For example, "I intend to take full control of my eating habits and to be kind and compassionate to myself." State your intention out loud at least three times per day.

Day Two: Make Sure That Your Thinking and Behaving Are in Alignment

Really be aware of where your thoughts are. If you think you shouldn't be eating something but are eating it anyway, keep in mind that you don't want to eat with guilty energy. Learn how to process what you are feeling quickly so that you are aware when you are "eating your emotions." If you are committed to acts of self-love, as yourself if you are behaving in ways that are more loving.

Day Three: What Behavior(S) Are You Willing to Let Go Of?

Write down what you are no longer willing to accept in your life. It could be how you allow others to treat you, or it could be how you allow yourself to treat you. Get ready to reclaim your life as you identify which behaviors are acceptable and which are not. Notice how many times you judge yourself. Write your thoughts here:

Day Four: Can You Tell the Difference between Physical Hunger and Emotional Hunger?

Learn how to ask yourself at various points during the day, "How am I feeling?" Face yourself with honesty. How observant can you be of what emotion you are feeling? Write your thoughts here:

Day Five: How Do You Sabotage Yourself When It Comes to Eating?

What are your food triggers, and how do you navigate them? What judgments and criticisms do you hear? What do you talk yourself into or out of? Journal your answers here:

Day Six: What Is Your Most Difficult Challenge Related to Food?

What situations do you find to be the biggest challenge to mindful eating? Is there a certain emotional trigger, time of day, or specific food in your pantry that presents the biggest challenge? Journal about what comes up for you:

Day Seven: How Do You Celebrate Your Little (or Big) Victories?

How can you be kinder to yourself and aware of your success? For example, perhaps you allowed yourself to choose one cookie, enjoyed it thoroughly, and found it to be enough (woo hoo!).

Gratitude

"Gratitude unlocks the fullness of life. It turns what we have into enough, and more. It turns denial into acceptance, chaos to order, confusion to clarity. It can turn a meal into a feast, a house into a home, a stranger into a friend. Gratitude makes sense of our paste, brings peace for today and creates a vision for tomorrow."

—Melody Beattie

Food for Thought: "Even-Ing Up the Pie"

Have you ever had this experience? You are standing in the kitchen or cleaning up the dining room table, and you are alone. The edges of the cake or pie (or casserole or a container of ice cream) are *uneven*. You pick up a fork and say, "Just one little nibble to *even it up*."

Mmm! It tastes so good—but look! It made the other side uneven. So again, you take the fork and dive in. And then again and again and again. A short while later, after you reemerge into consciousness, you realize you have eaten nearly the whole thing! So then you say, "Oh, what the heck?" And you finish it off.

Every time I share this experience at the Divine Dining Workshops, almost everyone in the room can relate! We have all had *unconscious* eating episodes and then "woken up" only to beat ourselves up for having been so weak.

It is amazing how our thoughts can lead us down this slippery slope. So here is a way to break that cycle: Next time you have the urge to "even up the pie," bring your full awareness to it. Ask yourself if it is what you truly want. If the answer is *yes*, then do it mindfully. Decide to take a sliver, and put it on a plate. Then sit down with it, bless it, and eat it while enjoying every bite.

Decisions, when made consciously and with *love* behind them, change the vibration and energy of how our bodies process what we eat.

Here are the five contemplations of food: take a moment before each meal to recite these contemplations.

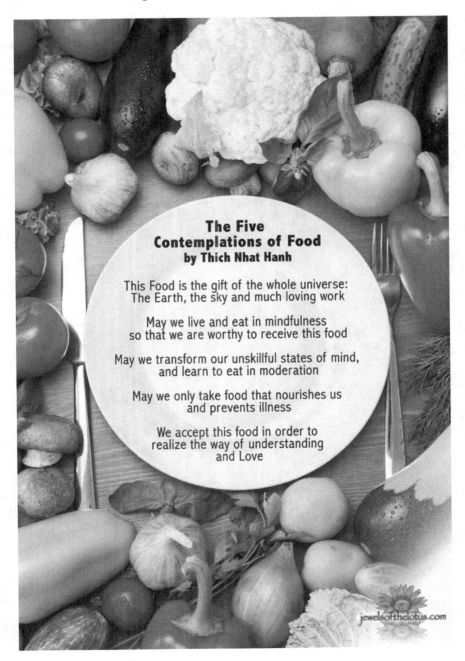

The Five Contemplations of Food
by Thich Nhat Hanh

This Food is the gift of the whole universe:
The Earth, the sky and much loving work

May we live and eat in mindfulness
so that we are worthy to receive this food

May we transform our unskillful states of mind,
and learn to eat in moderation

May we only take food that nourishes us
and prevents illness

We accept this food in order to
realize the way of understanding
and Love

jewelsofthelotus.com

9

The Divine Dining Method Twenty-One Day Plan

Introduction

Welcome to our twenty-one day guide to the Divine Dining Method!

Think of this exclusive guide as a supplement to our original seven-day Divine Dining Method workbook. The Divine Dining Method is about both the relationship you have with yourself and the relationship you have with your food. What you have in your hands is a guide to bring the divine into the sacred act of eating. When the twenty-one days are up and you've completed this guide, come back to revisit the process!

Each day, when you refer to this supplement, you'll read the affirmation, recommended crystal, inspirational quote, focus, journal prompt, and a recommended reading from the *Living Lotus* blog (https://www. livinglotusgroup.com/blogs/blog) to help you deepen the Divine Dining Method experience.

Finally, if you need further support, have any questions, or want to share your experiences and progress, you can email Catherine@livinglotusgroup. com or post in the private Facebook group made just for participants here: Divine Dining Life.

Remember, this is not a diet; it's a supreme act of self-love!

Wishing you divine dining!

Daily Meditation

Set aside five to ten minutes each day to meditate. Relax your body, and allow your breath to take you deeply within yourself. Ask your angels and guides to surround you with loving protection.

Bring your attention into your center and your awareness to the inner light that shines from within. Imagine your food addictions, struggles, and negative habits manifesting in front of you, and then see them released and dissolved by the divine light.

Ask your higher self to accompany you on your journey toward higher, healthier eating. Imagine that you are watching yourself from out of your body before you begin to eat. Pause before you begin to put the food into your mouth. Know that you can make positive food choices that nurture you.

Feel the energy within, and let it fill you. Inhale deeply. Exhale.

Know that you are always supported and loved by the divine.

Day One

One cannot think well, love well, sleep well, if one has not dined well.

—Virginia Woolf

Affirmation

"My eating habits can be healthy and nurturing."

Crystal

Today's crystal is clear quartz.

Focus

Set your intention and focus for the next twenty-one days. Get comfortable with holding the clear quartz in your meditation. Clear quartz helps bring clarity to the mind and release blockages. Take a deep breath. Make the commitment to yourself to approach food with a new attitude. This is the first powerful step toward freedom. Feel yourself align with this intention. Choose the words that feel right to you.

Journal

Record your meals and any thoughts that came to you during your morning meditation. What brought you to this course? How do you want to improve your relationship with food? Where are your struggles when it comes to eating? Is your struggle with eating too much or too little? Do you need to make better choices when it comes to *what, when,* or *how* you're eating?

Catherine Russo Epstein

Recommended Reading: Divine Dining

"Be one with the food." That is what I always tell my children when they are shoveling their dinner. Conscious eating is about being completely aware of the act of eating. It is not the shoveling or mindless stuffing of one's face. When we are fully engaged in the process of eating, we can deeply experience the tastes, sensations, and aromas of food. When you bring a conscious eating habit to your life, you'll be kinder to your digestive system, and you won't overeat. You'll be in tune with your body and stop when full. If you aren't ready to make the whole transformation of your eating habits, then try it with a snack or a light meal. Food can become a spiritual experience when it is approached from a mindful perspective.

Take a piece of dark, rich organic chocolate. Make sure you are sitting to do this (not leaning over the kitchen sink). Peel the wrapper back slowly, and take a deep breath.

Break off a small piece, and place it on your tongue. Let the flavor begin to fill your mouth with rapture. Slowly chew it. Let your awareness be on the sensations, taste, and motions.

As the chewing progresses and the chocolate begins to break down in your mouth, take another deep breath. You must truly savor this bite as it melts in your mouth before you have another bite.

Make this process a mindful meditation, and you will understand what it means to be one with the chocolate. Do this with all your meals, and you will be in full control of what you eat, how much you eat, and when you are sated. It is when we are "unconscious" that we inhale our food, only partially chewing, to fill that void in our lives.

Honor your hunger, and be sure to taste the flavors. Learn to wait for foods that will nourish your body and nurture your soul rather than reaching for the quick fix. Bless your food, and give thanks for it.

Breathe—and good eats!

42

Day Two

Change is the essence of life. Be willing to surrender what you are for what you could become.

—Reinhold Niebuhr

Affirmation

"I am open to change."

Crystal

Today's crystal is clear quartz.

Focus

Sometimes we may fall into a comfortable routine, allowing ourselves to get stuck in old habits and ways of living that may not be the healthiest or most positive. Content with comfort, we are resist change and the unknown rather than risk failure or vulnerability. But today is the day that you begin to open yourself up to *positive* change. Recognize your potential and all the possibilities in front of you.

Journal

Record your meals and any thoughts that came to you during your morning meditation. What do you want to change about yourself and your life? Focus on internal changes rather than external; be aware of all that you have and all that you are. What steps would you take to make these changes? What would they mean to you?

Recommended Reading: Rivers of Change

As you open to the waves of divine love that are flowing through the universe right now, remind yourself to tap into this flow. It can be easy to fall back into the old ways and to go into default mode, as we have lived that way for so long. It is important to stay vigilant about how you feel in any given moment.

With the planetary alignments, shifting consciousness, a new surge of hope, and countless other factors, what's an ordinary human to do?

There is no question that we are in the midst of radical changes. We are feeling them on an individual level, in community, and on a universal scale. Humanity is riding the wave of change, and our task is to be aware. Even when life gets intense, the best we can do for ourselves is to remain aware of our conditioned responses. This awareness is key and will lead us to make conscious choices to set ourselves free from the old—the old that keeps us bogged down.

"Awareness leads directly to understanding." A dear friend shared this with me, and it is true. Although sometimes I try to control my life and certain aspects of it, when I truly let go of the drama and expectations, I do find peace. This letting go is difficult for so many, but we know that holding on simply makes it more difficult. Learning to flow on the path leads toward freedom. The key is to *remember*. Remember to breathe, to love yourself, to be peaceful, and to just *be*.

We are purging so much old stuff right now, so keep reminding yourself that this is a release. Try not to get caught in the releasing energy; simply allow it to pass. We move forward as *one*! Together, let's let our lights shine as we ride on the rivers of change!

Peace and blessings to all.

Day Three

Self-love is the elixir of an immortal heart.

—Amy Leigh Mercree

Affirmation

"My relationship with food is positive."

Crystal

Today's crystal is clear quartz.

Focus

Too often we feel pressured into a certain "diet" or lifestyle change not for ourselves but to appear a certain way to others. When we do this, the focus shifts from health and happiness to insecurity and self-punishment. Know that food is not a vice to abstain from but a blessing to be enjoyed. Approach this program from a place of self-love. Your participation in the Divine Dining Method is less a means of self-discipline than a show of compassion toward yourself.

Journal

Record your meals and any thoughts that came to you during your morning meditation. What is your favorite meal to cook? Your favorite dessert to bake? Think about where your food has come from, and think about what certain foods mean to you. Taste and smell have powerful associations to emotional memories. Try to recall a memory in which you've shared a wonderful meal with great company. This will help change your attitude toward the food itself.

Recommended Reading: Can You Dare to be Yourself?

Have you ever believed in yourself and accomplished something you didn't think you could? Do you remember what that felt like? Exhilarating, perhaps? Imagination has no limits, so why should real life? Believe that you can do anything, and then stand back. Let your dreams unfold in amazing ways. Belief is an alignment within yourself, a linking of the head and the heart. It is the merging of all the energy that is you at your deepest core. It is the part of you that knows no limits or boundaries. If you can believe that anything is possible and feel that belief within your heart and soul, then you can reach the highest potential for your life. You can do anything! Take steps forward because, as you will learn, there are no mistakes—only lessons. Believe in yourself, your heart, and your life.

How authentic is your life? Where are you fully able to be yourself? What does being real mean to you? Authenticity means being aligned with our values. There is such freedom in an authentic life. As long as you are living in alignment with your core truth, anything that isn't in truth simply falls away.

Knowing what your values are and what is important to you is a individual process and one that is vital to any decision-making. What do you value? Do you value adventure, security, independence, contribution, family, and/or spirituality? The list goes on. Once you know how to prioritize your values, you can hone in on the choices that lie before you—and from there, you can make the decision with the highest potential.

Open yourself to the unlimited possibilities for your life! And answer this question: can you dare to be yourself?

Day Four

Listen to the inner light; it will guide you. Listen to inner peace; it will feed you. Listen to inner love; it will transform you, it will divinize you, it will immortalize you.

—Sri Chinmoy

Affirmation

"I am filled with the light and love of the divine."

Crystal

Today's crystal is rose quartz.

Focus

Rose quartz is a powerful yet gentle heart-healing stone. It allows us to open the heart so that we can receive and give more love; it also attracts loving energy. Set your intention today to flood your body with self-love and break the old patterns and conditionings that have held you back. Your only goal today is to bring pure love into the act of eating. When you focus on this act, your awareness fully illuminates all your senses. Open your heart center and see the love emanating from there. Let it envelope you and surround you with the divine.

Journal

Record your meals and any thoughts that came to you during your morning meditation. Set your intentions, as simple or as grand as they may be: What foods do you want to eat less of? What foods do you want to eat more of? What parts of yourself do you want to learn to love?

Recommended Reading: Benefits of the Divine Dining Method

What are the benefits of the Divine Dining Method? The Divine Dining Method is a conscious way to transform your mealtimes. By working with mindfulness, meditation, affirmations, and crystals, you will be guided to be more conscious and aware of your eating.

Here's a note by a recent participant: "The Divine Dining [Method] taught me to sit and relax while eating and to savor my food instead of rushing through a meal. I was often guilty of leaving the table mid-meal to write a note or put something away. Now I have been treating each meal as a sensory experience."

Many people ask me how the Divine Dining Method can help them. There are many benefits to this program. I'm so passionate about helping people make positive choices in their lives, including incorporating a mindfulness practice into the act of eating.

We all need to eat, right? If you've had issues with food (and who hasn't?), you might find the following list of benefits to be helpful.

Here are some of the benefits. First, the Divine Dining Method aids with weight management. This is not a diet; it's a supreme act of self-love that teaches us to be kinder to ourselves. Second, the Divine Diving Method works in conjunction with any eating style. Remember, it is the intention we put behind the act of eating that is most important. Third, the Divine Dining Method activates a healthy digestive system. Chewing completely and thoroughly before you even swallow will help stir the digestive juices. Finally, the Divine Dining Method encourages you to be in full control of *what* you eat (making healthy choices), *when* you eat (noting times of day, whether you are between meals, etc.), and *why* you eat (watching for emotional eating).

The Divine Dining Method

Day Five

*When you know in your bones that your body is a sacred gift,
you move in the world with an effortless grace. Gratitude and
humility rise up spontaneously.*

—Debbie Ford

Affirmation

"I am grateful for my body."

Crystal

Today's crystal is rose quartz.

Focus

Often, in our quests to lose inches or pounds, flatten our stomachs, or trim down our thighs, we take our bodies for granted. We forget the miracles that our bodies perform daily: not only is your body constantly taking care of you and keeping you alive, but also it allows you to taste, touch, smell, hear, see, walk, jump, dance, and laugh! We must remind ourselves that our bodies are gifts—gifts that we must be thankful for. With diets and unnatural weight loss programs, we end up trying to fight our bodies and their natural instincts; with the Divine Dining Method, we are simply learning to treat our bodies with care and respect through mindful eating.

Journal

Record your meals and any thoughts that came to you during your morning meditation. Take note of all the times in the past hour, day, or even week that you wished your body looked differently, that you compared your body to someone else's, or that you criticized another person's body.

Turn those negative thoughts into positive affirmations. Recognize your gratitude for your body.

Recommended Reading: Gratitude Rocks!

How amazing it is to give a gift from the heart. When we give from this place, we ride the continuous flow of energy and feel it flowing back to us. Scientific studies have shown that one of the fastest ways to heal your heart is to be of service to others. And being of service comes in many forms.

We can be of service financially by donating to worthwhile causes. We can be of service by listening to a friend in need. We can be of service while praying, creating, and donating time, as well as in countless other ways. We can also be of service by showing others how we appreciate them by passing along a touchstone or reminder for them to carry.

One great way to show appreciation and gratitude for another is to give him or her a gratitude rock. A gratitude rock is a randomly chosen crystal that has energetic properties. Conveniently packaged, a gratitude rock (if you choose to buy one) comes with a card explaining the individual properties and another card explaining its pay-it-forward purpose.

The energy of the abundance of the universe stands behind the concept of gratitude rocks and helps remind you to be in flow with all of life. The premise is simple. Throughout your day, show your appreciation to someone by giving that person a gratitude rock. Tell the person that you are grateful for him or her and that the stone is intended to show appreciation. If you receive a stone, set your intention that it will serve as a reminder to stay mindful throughout the day. This includes speaking kindly, staying authentic, and being in the present moment.

While the gifting of gratitude rocks is not a new idea, it helps one tap into the flow of giving. Gratitude rocks are all about paying it forward. They are based on the idea of appreciation and of acknowledging others for touching our lives in some way. When we express our appreciation with something tangible, such as a gratitude rock, we honor the light in another person.

Day Six

To be beautiful means to be yourself. You don't need to be accepted by others. You need to accept yourself.

—Thich Nhat Hanh

Affirmation

"I am not afraid to love myself."

Crystal

Today's crystal is rose quartz.

Focus

We are constantly receiving messages from the media surrounding us that we are not good enough as we are—so much is this the case that it has become quite difficult to love ourselves *and* all our imperfections. It may feel even *more* difficult, among these messages, to admit and embrace your self-love! But to love oneself truly *is* the greatest love of all, and we have to remember to treat ourselves kindly.

Journal

Record your meals and any thoughts that came to you during your morning meditation. Because today's focus is all about loving ourselves, make a list of fifteen things about yourself that you *love*. Think about inner *and* outer traits, as an exercise in loving and accepting ourselves, wholly.

Recommended Reading: Gratitude and Gold

Living as our authentic selves, we make choices based on what feels right to us rather than on what others think or what we think we are supposed to do. Our decision-making process is evolving to a state where we combine discernment, awareness, and love to sift through myriad inputs. This is all about staying clear in our emotions, thoughts, and energy fields. Being mindful of our creative process at all times will help manifest a more abundant life. We know that focusing on beauty and gratitude will bring more of that to us. Conversely, the energy that goes into worry or fear will create more of that too, so focus your energy on love and support, and allow more of that into your life!

Being aware of your thoughts (and the space before your thoughts) at all times will help hone your creative skills. We are powerful and skilled at manifesting lives beyond our wildest dreams! The energy of lack and limitation can go behind out thoughts and muck up our creations. How we feel about ourselves, any judgments we may have, and lingering doubts and limitations will all propel forward into the creative mix. It is with these extraneous thoughts and baggage that sometimes our creations are less than desirable.

It takes courage to face the world within and to be grateful for even the tough lessons. Being along for this ride and being fully focused on one's growth is no easy task. You always have choice. It is best to make your choices with full awareness. As Yoda once said, "Do or do not; there is no try."

What is imperative to remember in the creative process is that your thoughts and beliefs are what attract your situations to you, so if you have limiting thoughts or beliefs from an old paradigm, that is what your creation will be borne from. In other words, what you attract will be the sum of all of you—whether consciously or not. This is why releasing all old patterns, etc., is so important. Even little gaps in how you perceive your reality can manifest in less than stellar creations. You don't want your creations looking like Swiss cheese. Part of conscious creation is coming from your whole self. Discernment is a powerful part of your essence. It helps you tap into the inner radar in your core. Learn to trust yourself and what your body is telling you. Looking at life from the view of your higher self means that all of a sudden, the seemingly impossible drops away. You know you are a powerful being of divine, radiant light.

Keys to get to the gold essence within include

- ✓ honing our ability to discern truth from illusion;
- ✓ making choices from the heart;
- ✓ being mindful of our thoughts;
- ✓ staying in the flow of gratitude and love at all times;
- ✓ looking inward with grace and acceptance;
- ✓ forgiving ourselves for any perceived mistakes;
- ✓ knowing what distractions are pulling us off center; and
- ✓ creating from a place of stillness rather than frenzy.

So let's all go for the *gold*! Dive deep into the waters of your beautiful heart, resonate with gratitude, and move forward in pure, golden heart love. When your heart flows with gratitude, peacefulness prevails in your heart and all is right in your world!

Day Seven

You are very powerful, provided you know how powerful you are.

—Yogi Bhajan

Affirmation

"I am in alignment with my higher purpose."

Crystal

Today's crystal is yellow calcite.

Focus

Yellow calcite allows us to open to joy. When you are aligned with the divine will, you are in flow with the highest of all good. Calcite helps to release blockages in the solar plexus so that more of your true divine self can shine through. Yellow calcite helps the solar plexus, which deals with our sense of self, and gently opens it, allowing us to be who we are in a healthy way.

Journal

Record your meals and any thoughts that came to you during your morning meditation. Answer this question: if you could do anything, what would you do? Now answer this: what's holding you back from doing just that? We don't often realize how much we hold *ourselves* back from pursuing our goals and chasing our dreams. When you start to see your*self* differently, you'll start to see your world and your life differently. Follow your higher purpose.

Recommended Reading: Living Life on Your Own Terms—From Powerless to Powerful (Three Ways to Regain Your Power)

One question: are you living life on your own terms? As you ponder the answer, think about what "on your own terms" means to you.

We all want to feel in control of our own destinies, but how many of us feel stuck in the rut of same old, same old? Are you ready to reclaim your power and enjoy living life on your *own* terms?

In my own life and in the lives of people I work with, it is sometimes hard to get out of the cycle of complacency. You get comfortable, and maybe you feel a stirring of discontent, but it isn't really enough to stand up and shake it off. You may feel a bit off-kilter but can't identify its source. You are living each day by tending to the tasks of surviving, but are you really living? Take a moment to sit with these questions and then listen to your answers.

Transformation doesn't have to be the "hit by the cosmic two-by-four" kind of change. We've all had that at some point, and it can be quite an upheaval. We've all heard the nudges and whispers of the inner self, and we've ignored it or made excuses. Then *wham*! We get whacked by the "cosmic two-by-four" to force change upon us. The good news is that it doesn't have to be so dramatic. Sometimes just one small step can move us in the right direction. Doesn't that sound more palatable than change being forced on us?

Since I like to keep things simple (breathe in) and easy (breathe out), the place to start is with a renewed commitment to getting back in control and to leading a more heart-centered life. If you've taken a more resigned approach and think that you can't make the changes you want, think again.

Here are the steps that show you how to move from feeling powerless to feeling powerful! I share these steps with my clients, and I use them in my own life!

Commitment

Renew your commitment to your life and your journey. When you accept where you are right now, it helps bring your awareness back to the present. Accept the feeling or emotion that is up for you, and check in with your body. From this point, you can take stock of what is in your life and identify what can stay and what needs to go. Accepting and not resisting can help take you to the next step. Give yourself permission to change.

Clarity

The next step is to get clear on where you want to go. What is it that you want? Sit down with your journal and make a list of ten or more words or qualities that make you feel alive again. For example, you might write *compassionate, peaceful, joyful, old, caring, present, energetic,* or *courageous.* You get the idea. Once you've identified the top ten, narrow your list to the three that speak to your soul the most. Don't think about the right answer; rather, allow what is in your heart at this moment to reveal itself. View the situation from a higher perspective so you can regain the feeling of being empowered. Feel all your energy returning back to your core. This must happen before you can focus on what to do next. Once you've identified your three words, set your intention to embody these traits. Now write them on an index card. Although these change often for me, my overriding words are *awake, aware,* and *alive.* What are your words?

Connection

Now that you have reconnected with your highest and best self, the vision for your life can begin to unfold. This is the third step, but by no means is it the final one. After you've pulled in all your energy, you are now ready to listen more fully to the inner callings of your soul. No more excuses or denials; firmly commit to regaining your *power.* After you've made the connection, just ask for guidance for the next step. Trust that it will unfold for you, and then follow the stirrings of your heart.

Once you *recommit* to yourself, *clarify* your vision again, and *reconnect* to your best self to regain your power, you will send a message to the universe that you are ready. Taking these steps will help you live life on your own terms!

Day Eight

You must maintain a state of happiness, a state of joy to let the positive thoughts emanate from your mind ... If you are in a state of joy, your thoughts emanate positive energy."

—Girdhar Joshi

Affirmation

"I am filled with pure life energy."

Crystal

Today's crystal is yellow calcite.

Focus

Working with yellow calcite guides us in supporting and nurturing ourselves. Remember to take care of yourself and to treat yourself with kindness and respect in your actions *and* your thoughts. When we are comfortable with ourselves and act from a place of love instead of fear, *that* is when we can bring about great changes in our lives. In these great changes, we can find great joy!

Journal

Record your meals and any thoughts that came to you during your morning meditation. Make the conscious effort today to smile. When you are in your car or at your desk or doing the dishes, take time to notice your facial expression. If it's not a smile, turn it into one. Even the simple act of grinning can bring joy to your heart. Make another conscious effort to put a smile on someone else's face. Write about your experiences.

Recommended Reading: Jumpstart Your Joy!

Take time this month to celebrate the heart in all its glory! The heart has the ability to stay open during sadness, joy, friendship, listening to a friend, and connecting with a child. The heart has the capacity to be strong yet vulnerable, soft yet tough, grateful, and accepting. Keep it open, keep it loving, and keep it radiant!

When we open our hearts and give from our true authentic selves, something magical happens. We allow our true divine radiance to flow through us, and as it does, it heals and transforms us. In turn, it heals and transforms those around us. The true nature of giving arises not *from*, but *through* us. Thus, the flow of energy becomes a beautiful stream of light in which we can immerse ourselves and therefore allow our true radiance to shine out.

Choosing to give from our hearts means letting go of what we expect in return. It means truly living in the moment and allowing the act of giving to be the point. In doing this, our hearts can open like the lotus flower.

We are all on this journey together. May we breathe in peaceful, loving kindness, and may all be free together.

Jumpstart your joy! Go forth, remembering to shine your light to others. Remember that with each day, and each moment, you have the ability to create yourself anew. Stand fully in your own power and be the example. Make your life a sacred event with every thought, action, and interaction. Life was meant to be fully experienced, the bitter and the sweet. Enjoy every drop.

It's time. Jumpstart your joy!

Day Nine

Plant your own garden and decorate your own soul, instead of waiting for someone to bring you flowers.

—Veronica A. Shoffstall

Affirmation

"I have the power to make positive change."

Crystal

Today's crystal is yellow calcite.

Focus

Think about the changes you want to make in your life. Go beyond food: perhaps you'd like to begin a spiritual practice, take an art class, read a certain number of books, or keep a cleaner home or car or office space. Who is the ideal version of yourself? What does she do that you don't? What does a day in her life look like? What's keeping you from becoming her?

Journal

Record your meals and any thoughts that came to you during your morning meditation. In your focus today, you have been concentrating on the changes you'd like to see in your life. Many times, those changes become wishes accompanied by an "If only ..."—we say, "I'd meditate daily, if only there were a few more hours in a day." Or, "I'd take a painting class, if only I could find someone to go with me." Or, "I'd have a cleaner home, if only I had the money for a housekeeper." Now eliminate that "if only" train of thought on the page and in your mind. The power is all yours to become the person you want to be.

Recommended Reading: What Is Your Vision?

What is your vision for the new earth? What are you focused on? Where are your thoughts right now? Do you believe that it is possible to manifest what we desire—in freedom and in joy? Is it possible to imagine living in a world with like-minded souls supporting and nurturing one another—where there is harmony and love, passion and joy? The answer is to start now by transforming your life as it is in this moment. Embracing yourself in all your human glory is the best place to begin.

As many spiritual teachers will tell you, the way to transform your life is by reaching the inner world through awareness. All you need do is tap into it. But with the intensity of energies increasing on this planet over the past few months, coupled with personal and global dramas, how do we really find that center? We find it by entering the present moment and knowing the peace we so long for resides there. If we allow ourselves to be calm and still, even if only for a moment, we can find peace even during the storm.

Our challenge is to truly observe and be the witness to our behaviors, ideally while interacting with others. When you can view yourself from this higher perspective and integrate all the parts of you that are participating, you gain the ability to allow the drama to unfold without getting caught in it. This will help you identify the emotions that are brought up without being sucked in. Doing this allows us to continue to disengage from the story and to be present for our own process.

Enter into stillness as often as you are able. Open to your own divinity and thereby transform your world. Enter into stillness via your heart, join with your higher self, and together we can transform the planet!

What is your vision? Believe it, and create it!

Day Ten

We delight in the beauty of the butterfly, but rarely admit the changes it has gone through to achieve that beauty.

—Maya Angelou

Affirmation

"I choose new and nurturing ways to nourish my body."

Crystal

Today's crystal is carnelian.

Focus

Carnelian works on clearing out blockages at an emotional level, helping to strengthen the second chakra, and releasing any old patterns or addictions. We process so much of the world around us in the second chakra, which is where addictive and possibly harmful patterns form. We must clear out these old patterns, and we must create space for new and healthy habits to come into our lives.

Journal

Record your meals and any thoughts that came to you during your morning meditation. Think about your routines and your habits. What do you do each morning? Where in your day can you make space for new, positive ways to spend your time? Now consider your habits—not only your physical habits (snacking late, nail-biting, smoking), but also your emotional habits. Think about who you surround yourself with and about how you tend to treat people. Clear out habits that no longer serve you or others.

Recommended Reading: Life Begins at the End of Your Comfort Zone

Ponder those words for a moment: "life begins at the end of your comfort zone." What do they mean to you? Is your life a dance between the old and the new, excitement and fear, or caution and recklessness?

Are you able to take a leap without taking a dive?

How many of us play it safe as we listen to the nagging voice inside? The voice tells us to stay small or quiet, as we might not be good enough, we might not succeed, or we might make a mistake. Well, we've all been there, and it is a human trait to stay with what is safe and comfortable. How do you know when it is time to follow your heart? Learning about yourself and the inner workings of your heart is a deep process. It is also a process that can be rewarding and that helps you shed the other voices that have accumulated over your lifetime.

What is it that pulls at your heartstrings? How can you get out of the box that has been so neatly wrapped up as your life? I recently took an art workshop, and I was extremely uncomfortable and stiff. The other people were creating with many different media and having fun. I was so uptight, wanting to create something pretty, that I was frozen. After it ended, I went home and cried. Was it the voice of the "stay inside the lines" critic? Or was that I didn't want to put myself out there? Weeks later I found a book, *The Tao of Watercolor*, that helped me unleash the pent-up artist within. This book helped me realize that there is no perfection in art; no one is standing over me judging me. So now, when I have time, I sit down and create. It flows, sometimes easier than other times. But I now have fun with the process.

So isn't it time you give your inner critic the day off? Or better yet, let the critic go. Acknowledge that it is okay to *be*. Simply becoming aware of how many times we judge ourselves in the course of a lifetime is staggering! Be your own best friend and cheerleader. Let your heart's emotions lead the way, and follow the path. Check in with your inner self often. The best way to stretch your comfort zone is to take small steps—try different types of classes, take a different route to work, take singing lessons, start a home business, be like a kid again, and be joyful.

Get to know yourself on a deep level. Know your heart, and learn about your emotions inside and out. Free yourself from any guilt or shame or feelings of low self-worth. It's time now to stand fully in your own power and not to be afraid to show your stuff! This is not about the limitations of the ego but the freedom of the heart and soul. You are ready! Put one foot in front of the other, and let the wind and river carry you in the flow of divine energy. Be solid in your core and true to your heart! Be peace in action, and know that it really is okay to color outside the lines—in fact, art is like life: it is more about the process than the end result. As your heart opens, ask yourself these two deep questions:

✓ Are you connecting with joy in your life?
✓ Are you sharing your light to bring joy to others?

Get up, get out, and dance! Know that it is safe and beautiful just outside your comfort zone. There is much to be experienced and much life to be *lived*.

❧

Day Eleven

I would maintain that thanks are the highest form of thought;
and that gratitude is happiness doubled by wonder.

—G.K. Chesterton

Affirmation

"I recognize that food is a blessing, for which I am thankful."

Crystal

Today's crystal is carnelian.

Focus

Turn your attention to your grocery list. Food shopping, preparation, and eating should be joyful tasks. Do not resign grocery shopping to the tedium of everyday life: treat it as a fresh slate and a new opportunity to make mindful, healthy choices. Remember to shop with your conscious mind, *not* your impulsive stomach! Purchase foods that will be kind to your body. Remember that snacking does not have to be a guilty pleasure: healthy and tasty are not mutually exclusive!

Journal

Record your meals and any thoughts that came to you during your morning meditation. Take some time to research some recipes that interest you—whether you want to incorporate more vegan food into your diet, make healthy snacks to munch on, or switch up your breakfast routine, there are numerous food blogs and websites for inspiration. Start collecting these recipes in your journal, and choose two or three per week to try. Make cooking creative and enjoyable!

Recommended Reading: Life Gems

<u>Here are some rules to live by:</u>

- ✓ Count your blessings (even and especially when it's tough).
- ✓ Go above and beyond what's expected of you. (Go the extra mile.)
- ✓ Don't quit. (Turn your mistakes into lessons.)
- ✓ Look for the good in everyone you meet. (Share your best self.)
- ✓ Focus on the positive. (Be aware of your thoughts.)
- ✓ Be humble. (Let your actions speak louder than your words.)
- ✓ Treat every day as if it's a gift. (Use it wisely.)
- ✓ Clear away clutter, and end distractions. (Spend your time wisely.)
- ✓ Live every day as if it were your last. (What would you do differently?)
- ✓ Treat all people as if they matter (and make eye contact).
- ✓ Laugh at yourself and life. (Be lighthearted.)
- ✓ Attend to the details. (Don't neglect the little things.)
- ✓ Be focused on the bigger picture. (Hold the highest vision for your life.)
- ✓ Greet every day with a smile. (Say *thank you* when you first wake up.)
- ✓ Be focused on the bigger picture or goal. (Take one day at a time.)
- ✓ Don't allow negativity to pull you down. (Guard your energy.)
- ✓ Search for the seed of goodness. (Look for the positive in any situation.)
- ✓ Happiness and peace lie within you (so find it and nurture it).
- ✓ Be patient (as nothing external can have any power over you).
- ✓ Always be larger than your problems. (Believe in your abilities.)
- ✓ Live simply.
- ✓ Take time for yourself every day (even if it is just five minutes).

Day Twelve

One of the very nicest things about life is the way we must regularly stop whatever we are doing and devote our attention to eating.

—Luciano Pavarotti

Affirmation

"I will be fully aware and joyful when eating."

Crystal

Today's crystal is carnelian.

Focus

It is hard to keep our attitudes toward food positive when eating becomes a struggle for control, but we must remember that there is joy in cooking, tasting, and sharing meals with our loved ones, and eating does not always have to be an inner battle. Some of the best memories are shared around a dinner table!

Journal

Record your meals and any thoughts that came to you during your morning meditation. Since today is all about the love of food, let's plan a dinner party—imaginary or otherwise! Pick ten guests. Take care in planning your favorite meals to make: some appetizers, an entrée, and a dessert. Choose nutritious and delicious recipes that require the freshest ingredients. If you can, send a few invites out!

Recommended Reading: Twelve Ways to Bring Mindfulness to Everyday Life

Mindfulness is the social buzzword these days. Everyone seems to be talking about how it is important to be more mindful in our lives. There are many studies that prove its effectiveness. The concept of mindful living has even made the cover of major magazines! Intuitively, we know mindfulness can make a difference in how we relate to ourselves and to others. We also recognize that it is easier to be mindful when we are in a yoga class with other peaceful souls; there is soft music playing, and we are steadfastly focused on holding a pose. But the real test of our *mindful mettle*, so to speak, is this question: How do we bring that awareness into our lives if we work in a negative office or when the traffic is bad, people are cranky, the phone is ringing, and the baby is crying? The short answer is to *pay attention* to what is present in this moment.

What is mindfulness? Just think of this simple definition: mindfulness is focused awareness of the present moment without judgment. Here are some ways to bring mindfulness into everyday life. (Hint: read each one with full awareness.)

1) *Bring loving awareness* to the present moment by stopping what you are doing, drawing in a deep breath, and being aware of how you are feeling.
2) *Develop the capacity* to pay attention to the moment.
3) *Learn to listen to your inner voice* and follow your intuition (learn the difference between the inner voice (positive and loving) and the inner critic (negative and harsh).
4) *Take care of the future* by being in the present.
5) *Develop insight* into your own process by being compassionate.
6) *Be a vehicle or conduit* so that powerful and loving energy flows through you. (And being in touch with the present moment enough to feel this energy.)
7) *Be aware of your thoughts, feelings, and emotions* in any given moment without judgment.

8) *Pause, ponder, and then proceed*: take a moment and a breath before responding. This is especially helpful in an conversation.

9) *Practice being comfortable in the uncomfortable.*

10) *Live with acceptance* of this moment (no matter what is occurring).

11) *Learn to view the world from a place of gratitude*, even being grateful for your challenges, as they are contributing to your growth. (See the beauty in all your life.)

12) *Bring conscious awareness to conversations* with others (learn to listen intently, without being focused on what you're going to say next).

Day Thirteen

Growth itself contains the germ of happiness.

—Pearl S. Buck

Affirmation

"I celebrate my growth and allow what is best for me."

Crystal

Today's crystal is aventurine.

Focus

Aventurine is a heart-healing stone that works gently with our emotions. It soothes and calms, serving to remind us of how far we have come. Continue celebrating how far you have come, and allow yourself to feel your growth. Allow your heart to fill with the joy and beauty from within. Acknowledge the work you've done so far, and let that feeling of pride dance in and around you.

Journal

Record your meals and any thoughts that came to you during your morning meditation. Use today to reflect on your progress thus far in the Divine Dining Method. Where have you noticed changes in your feelings toward food and in your feelings toward yourself? Where have you noticed setbacks or negativity? What do you still hope to accomplish? Set an intention for the remainder of the program, with the awareness that the process of mindful eating is an ongoing journey that we must learn to enjoy and approach from a place of love.

Recommended Reading: Believe It or Not, the Choice Is Yours

Change your beliefs, and change your life! What beliefs do you currently hold about yourself? Are you a strong, loving, and wonderful human being with many gifts to share? Or do you believe that you can never get what you want or are deeply unlovable? What do you hold up as true for yourself?

Sometimes these beliefs are held deep within, and learning about them can give us answers as to why we sabotage ourselves in life. Maybe we feel we are not good enough, smart enough, or pretty enough, and we incorporate these beliefs into our own beings. These are beliefs we may have acquired along the way, having heard them from critical voices or from those who had their own fears. These beliefs are not true to our core essences.

Now is the time to review the deep beliefs you hold and to reclaim the ones that are true. You are a loving, beautiful being with many gifts to share, and all you need to reclaim that power is to stay true to your vision. When you feel yourself dropping into the abyss of self-recrimination, your task is to take notice and ask yourself what feels true to you. Emotions are the key that will point us to where we are not aligned, and we can learn to recognize quickly when this drop in energy happens. When we notice this drop, being aware of our truth can bring us back into alignment. Simply ask yourself if it is true for you that you are not worthy. Step back into the higher plane of empowered receptivity. Look out at your life from the truth—and own it fully. Use your vision to become inspired to create.

What is your inspired vision? And what gifts can you freely share with the world? Can you be the visionary of the future? Take the next moment to think of what gifts you can share with the world—the innate gifts that you can give freely. Maybe you can give a loving heart, beautiful artwork, touching poetry, an awesome smile, a majestic garden, your courage, deep joy, an intuitive ear, or joyous music and lyrics. Perhaps the gift of your life story will help others to overcome similar challenges. Consider the gift born of a deep desire to make this world a far better place for our children and their children.

This is the time to make a plan to plant a new belief system! Plant trees, plant seeds, plant your desires, water them with deep love, and watch what blooms.

Believe it or not—the choice is yours!

Day Fourteen

Cooking demands attention, patience, and above all, a respect for the gifts of the earth. It is a form of worship, a way of giving thanks.

—Judith B. Jones

Affirmation

"I will treat preparing, eating, and enjoying my food as sacred acts."

Crystal

Today's crystal is aventurine.

Focus

Today, if possible, cook your own breakfast, lunch, or dinner. Take time and care in preparing your meals. Do not rush through any steps in this preparation; when it comes time to sit and eat, do so in a sacred space. Eliminate any distractions. Focus completely on the meal. Be fully present, experiencing the meal with all your senses.

Journal

Record your meals and any thoughts that came to you during your morning meditation. Food preparation and cooking can be acts of creativity. Describe each step in making your meals today as an exercise in being fully aware of your actions. Acknowledge the gratitude within for the ability to cook, eat, and enjoy the food.

Recommended Reading: Re-Minding: The Gifts of a Mindfulness Practice

How often do you sit and observe your thoughts? We all have been reading and learning about how being more mindful can help us reduce stress and improve our relationships and interactions with others. There are many articles about how to develop a daily meditation practice. There are so many different ways to meditate, and one of my favorites is mindfulness meditation. Mindfulness can be defined as "observing your thoughts, feelings, and emotions without judgment."

If you can sit and practice for at least ten minutes daily by simply being aware and observing, without judging the process, you will find it becomes easier to practice over time.

In Jon Kabat-Zinn's book, *Letting Everything Become Your Teacher*, the chapter on "re-minding" says it all: "Given all the momentum behind our doing, getting ourselves to remember the preciousness of the present moment seems to require somewhat unusual and even drastic steps. This is why we make a special time each day for formal meditation practice. It is a way of stopping, a way of 're-minding' ourselves, of nourishing the domain of being for a change. It's a way of 're-bodying' too."

As I share with my coaching clients, the most important thing is not to empty the mind and have no thoughts. The most important key to remember in a meditation practice is how you treat yourself when thoughts come up. In other words, *be aware of your thoughts, but don't judge yourself for having them.*

Take some time each day to give your being the gift of "re-minding."

Day Fifteen

At its most essential, the apple you hold is a manifestation of the wonderful presence of life ... It feeds our body, and if we eat it mindfully, it also feeds our soul and recharges our spirit.

—Thich Nhat Hanh

Affirmation

"I will engage all my senses during each meal to be fully present through the act of eating."

Crystal

Today's crystal is aventurine.

Focus

Simply bringing a little mindfulness to the table can help you realize that food doesn't have to have power over you. That same mindfulness will also help you enjoy your meal a little more by helping you concentrate wholly on every bite. The sensory experience of food is lost when we are in a rush to eat or are concentrating on what we should and shouldn't be eating. Devote your full attention to the meal!

Journal

Record your meals and any thoughts that came to you during your morning meditation. Just as we described the steps of preparation and cooking yesterday, today we will describe the experience of eating each meal. What did each meal smell like? Look like? Taste like? In this social media world, where people are *always* taking pictures of their food, take a sensory photo of it. Remember every detail. Eat with total mindfulness.

Recommended Reading: Peace Is Your Choice

Can you feel the joy that is within your heart? Sit for a moment, and breathe.

Can you feel the love that is all around you? Let the energy flow.

Can you sense the magic that lies within? Don't "think" about it.

Take a stand in your life, be upright, and be courageous. You can do it!

Believe that the heart is open to love to its full capacity whatever is winging its way toward you. Believe with all your might!

Accept with *grace* all that is in your life right now. Love it, and don't fight it. Peace is your choice—always *your* choice. It's your life and your choice.

Day Sixteen

At bottom, the heart that seeks to awaken, to live genuinely, is more real than anything.

—Ezra Bayda

Affirmation

"I live as my true and authentic self."

Crystal

Today's crystal is selenite.

Focus

Selenite helps us integrate our higher selves into the physical plane, bringing in the purest divine light. This link to your higher self will help you continue tuning into your body and what it needs. Be energized by your breath and the nourishing food you are blessed with. Connect to your inner wisdom, and live as your truest, most authentic self.

Journal

Record your meals and any thoughts that came to you during your morning meditation. Consider the times in your life when, in trying to please others, you sacrificed your truest self. What has led you to do that? Is it in eating a certain way, or in your attitude toward food? Does it manifest in the way you treat yourself? Create a connection between your truest inner self and your outer self. Let the true *you* shine through at all times.

Recommended Reading: Seven Ways to Live on Purpose

Are you living your life on purpose? Or is life just happening to you, just winging through your day?

It is amazing to me how many people still feel they aren't important. In my coaching practice, I am passionate about helping people reconnect with themselves! It's all about reconnecting with your higher purpose and offering your gifts to the world.

It's time to own your power and who you are—time to share your gifts with the world! And let's be honest here. Isn't it time you made friends with yourself again?

Seven Ways to Live on Purpose

<u>Self-acceptance</u>. Be aware of how you speak to yourself. Even self-deprecating talk can be damaging. Learn to observe your thoughts and actions without judging. Your life has been a series of challenges and deep lessons that have all brought you to where you are right now. Accept all of it! Fully!

Creative Expression. Within every person is a need to express. How do you tap into that which wants to be expressed in your life? Think about where your passions lie and reconnect with them. Whatever makes you fully come to life is your connection to your higher purpose. Get back in touch with whatever that is for you, and go out and do it!

Let go of what holds you back. Get to know your own energy. Learn to identify who or what lifts you up in life, and identify who or what drags you down. While sometimes you can't avoid all negative people or situations in your life, you can learn to let it pass through you without letting it stick to you. It's time to clear your energy!

Revitalize. Stop complaining that you don't have time for yourself. (I know, I know.) There is only *one* way to get time to recharge: give yourself permission. Studies of the most successful and busiest people are showing that they make time for meditation—at least twenty minutes per day. I know a woman who was overwhelmed and didn't think she could commit, so she started with three minutes per day. She found it so helpful that she gradually worked her way up to twenty minutes and is still doing it over one year later.

Mind your thoughts. Be diligent about your thoughts. Humans think fifty thousand to seventy thousand thoughts per day! (And it's not all about what's for dinner.) Be aware of the "tapes" you replay over and over again, but also know that you can insert new tapes. Neuroscience teaches us that we can retrain our brains. (Google neuroplasticity and scientific studies.) You can learn a new way to think, but like everything else, it takes practice, commitment, and persistence!

Live authentically. Be true to yourself once again. Reacquaint yourself with all the yearnings of your soul. Reawaken to your true self. Let go of doing things out of obligation, and start doing things again from enthusiasm. I know you have the ability to move beyond your fears. You have the courage to fully live again!

Follow your passion. I know your passion is to feel reconnected to your life and to once again feel awake, aware, and alive. Find the spark again that fuels the fire of your desires. Remember that when you live more fully from your heart, you affect the lives of those all around you. Whoever you come in contact with will feel that something special from you, and it will help others rise to be their best selves.

Don't ever think that you are too small or insignificant to make a difference. Make a ripple in your own pond. Play your part in the healing of the world!

Day Seventeen

What is always speaking silently is the body.

—Norman Brown

Affirmation

"I will listen to my body, and find what feels good for me."

Crystal

Today's crystal is selenite.

Focus

Mindful eating is a chance to listen to our bodies. It is a chance to know what makes our bodies feel good, when our bodies are full, and what doesn't agree with us. Mindful practices, such as yoga and meditation, also keep us in tune with our bodies by helping us develop a mindful presence that we carry with us in the world. Listen more closely to your body and the way it reacts to certain foods and eating habits. When you find what feels good—not just instant gratification but long-term satisfaction—that's when you are moving forward on your way to sustain a healthy lifestyle.

Journal

Record your meals and any thoughts that came to you during your morning meditation. After each meal, take a few minutes to sit in silence and scan the body. Do you feel overwhelmingly full? Are you still hungry? Does your food feel nourishing and fresh, or does it make your stomach feel uneasy? Take some time throughout the day to scan your body as well. What are you feeling in each part of it, from head to toe?

Recommended Reading: Enter into Stillness

I know what you're thinking: *I can't turn off my brain, I don't have the time,* or *I've tried it, and it doesn't work for me.*

Resistance shows up in the strangest ways—especially when it comes to something that we know is good for us. If we understand the benefits of having a meditation practice, why do we resist it? Although I can't answer that specific question, I can tell you that my belief is that there is *no wrong way to meditate.* And, keeping that in mind, what if I told you that there is a surefire way to reduce stress, reduce anxiety, and bring more peace, focus, and happiness into your life? What if I told you that it can be done by committing to only several minutes per day? Would you believe me?

Before I founded Living Lotus Group, and long before I became a meditation teacher, I experimented with many different forms of meditation. In all my years of study, and after many frustrating attempts, I've finally found techniques that work best for me and for the many clients I serve. I developed a meditation program called "Enter into Stillness" as a way of helping people get reacquainted with themselves so that they can become more balanced and focused.

There is an old adage that says, "People who say they have no time to meditate are the ones who need it the most." This is my life's work: Not only do I *love* to help people explore their inner worlds, but I also help them appreciate and accept what they find there.

With all the distractions and drama, it is difficult not to get caught up in what is happening around us—yet this is when we need to maintain our centered calmness.

As many spiritual teachers will tell you, the way to transform your life is by reaching the inner world through awareness. All you need is to tap into it, but with the intensity of energies increasing on this planet over the past few months, coupled with personal and global dramas, how do we really find that center? We do so by entering the present moment and knowing that the peace we so long for resides there. If we allow ourselves to be calm and still, even if only for a moment, we can find peace, even during the storm.

Our challenge is to truly observe and be the witness of our behaviors, ideally while interacting with others. When you can view yourself from this higher perspective and integrate all the parts of yourself that are participating, you gain the ability to allow the drama to unfold without getting caught in it, as discussed previously. This help you identify the emotions that are brought up without being sucked in. Doing this allows you to continue to disengage from the story and to be present for your own process.

Enter into stillness as often as you are able. Open to your own divinity and thereby transform your world. Enter into stillness through your heart.

Benefits of Meditation

Meditation:

- reduces stress and anxiety,
- increases mental focus,
- strengthens the immune system, and
- reconnects us with our hearts.

Not only will entering into stillness help you explore your inner world, but it will also help you actually learn to appreciate and accept what you find there!

Day Eighteen

When I let go of what I am, I become what I might be. When I let go of what I have, I receive what I need.

—Lao Tzu

Affirmation

"I will acknowledge, accept, and release my struggles with food."

Crystal

Today's crystal is selenite.

Focus

Change can be scary, overwhelming, or risky. We grow comfortable with the way things are, even if we are unhappy, because we adapt and tolerate situations over time. But now is the time to make positive changes! That doesn't have to mean letting go of your favorite indulgences forever, but instead of eating a bagel every single day, eat it once a week; instead of having two scoops of ice cream, stick with one. Letting go is not absolute; the goal is to develop a practice of mindfulness that will allow you to fully enjoy the food you eat without thinking of it as a "guilty" pleasure or feeling as though you are starving yourself to control portions.

Journal

Record your meals and any thoughts that came to you during your morning meditation. Think about your entire life, considering your habits, your material possessions, your relationships, and your routines. What can you let go of? What can you clear out? Sometimes the physical act of cleaning out and organizing will motivate and inspire you to let go and "spring clean" both your inner and outer worlds. Set aside time to clean out a particular closet or room in your home. Give away or donate what you no longer need.

Recommended Reading: Sometimes Surrender Is the Best Action

I've come to the realization lately that I can't control everything. No, really: I can't control it all, as much as I'd like to. Currently, the circumstances of my life are driving this point home to me—again and again. It's time for me to come into acceptance and surrender to the moment.

Take a look at your life right now. Where do you need to step back and surrender? Where can you stop trying to go against the current? "But, I'm not ready to give up," you say. This is not to say that you need to "give up," which has more of a fear-based component to it. When fear is the underlying force behind anything, the manifestation is less than stellar. It does mean that it is time to become larger than your problems and to see them already solved, and in miraculous ways. It means having a faith that is so strong it overrides anything in the outer appearance of your life. It means nurturing a healthy dose of trust: trust in yourself, trust in the universe, and trust that all will work out well.

Your life is your mission—and sometimes that means you need to let go of trying to control every step. Surrendering is a way of reinforce your belief in the ultimate magic of the universe. Surrendering is a bold act that takes guts and courage.

If you can only remember the true nature of the universe and that your life purpose is to awaken fully, you can step away from the everyday and reconnect with your highest self.

Let go of fear, doubt, and worry; they are drains on your energy. As I tell many of my life-coaching clients, "Resignation is giving up. Surrender is letting go." Feel the energetic difference between these two.

Take a closer look at your life now. What is it that you need to surrender? Believe that where you are right now is necessary for your soul growth and that this is all part of the larger plan. Breathe deep, and relax into the knowledge that all will be well.

Remember, sometimes surrendering is the best action.

Day Nineteen

Your heart is where your inner light resides. It is part of every sacred journey to reconnect with your inner light, step into your divinity, spread the light of love before you, return to the essence of love, and inspire others to do the same.

—Molly Friedenfeld

Affirmation

"The light of the divine shines within me."

Crystal

Today's crystal is hematite.

Focus

Hematite is a grounding and protective stone, one that is great for your circulatory system. It helps us remember that our words and actions affect everyone around us; it also reminds us of our divinity and our ability to shine our inner light. Allow your beauty and true self to radiate to the world.

Journal

Record your meals and any thoughts that came to you during your morning meditation. Focus on letting your inner light shine through by completing the following to-do list today:

1. Do something for yourself: take some time to create, watch your favorite movie, or treat yourself to a massage or manicure!

2. Do something for someone else: bake a favorite treat, call up a friend you haven't spoken to in a while, or send a "thinking of you" card.

3. Do something for the world: donate old clothes, sign up to volunteer, or even sign an online petition for a cause you care about!

Recommended Reading: The Fire in Your Heart!

This life isn't about accumulating "stuff"; it is about releasing (or burning off) all the things that hold you back from your true nature. It is the paradox of this life that it takes time to be what we already are.

We are all blessed with the beauty of a pure heart at birth, but living in this world and society creates pain and trauma. We slowly close up, build a wall, and retreat within. We avoid facing the muck—it feels too overwhelming.

Notice that if you were to stand in full appreciation for all your scars and lessons, that would change the way you feel about your story. Allow this awareness to permeate your thoughts, without judgment. When you notice the life force within and drink in the purity of the spirit, you notice that cleansing begins to take place. A sense of peace lies within, and as you stay with this peace, it begins to grow stronger and more palpable. As this peace comes into the foreground and you let go of things that once hurt, you begin to see the gifts of the lessons. You acknowledge the hurts, bless them, and then release them. It is in this release that we open to our true natures.

Today we take time to acknowledge the beauty and fragility of the heart. Feel the beat of your own heart as it merges with the heart of the earth. This inner drumbeat calls you forth. When you listen to the wisdom of the heart, it will tell you what it wants and what it needs. This is the time to be who you already are.

Day Twenty

The best way to capture moments is to pay attention. This is how we cultivate mindfulness. Mindfulness means being awake. It means knowing what you are doing.

—Jon Kabat-Zinn

Affirmation

"I will remain mindful throughout my day, especially during mealtimes."

Crystal

Today's crystal is hematite.

Focus

In clearing out the old energies within and creating space for change, you've made room for the new and amazing *you* to shine through. Allow your hematite to help you reflect your inner beauty. Be mindful of the way you feel toward yourself and others. Reprogram any negativity you detect in your energy; think only positive thoughts.

Journal

Record your meals and any thoughts that came to you during your morning meditation. Make the conscious choice to love yourself today. Give yourself some extra attention by staying mindful and fully *experiencing* your day, even the mundane parts of it. Think back on today, and record at least three memorable moments—moments you would have ordinarily overlooked had you not remained mindful. Remember that old cliché: every day is a gift!

Recommended Reading: Relax! Mindful Ways to Relieve Stress

What's your first reaction when someone tells you to relax or calm down? For some, their immediate response is, "I'm *not* tense!" Then their inner voice kicks in and says, "Yeah, maybe I'd better take it easy," and even though they might not want to show it, they let go just a bit.

Take a moment now and scan your body. Sometimes we are just plodding through our days without awareness of our physical states. We wonder why we feel so tired all the time. Learning to check in with our bodies is the fastest way to get back in touch with what we are feeling.

Stress is a pervasive part of our society. Simply walk down the street and observe the expressions on the faces of other folks. Or you might not even see their faces but the tops of their heads—as they look down at their phones.

Awareness is key. As a life coach, I always teach people that you can't make lasting changes if you aren't aware of the issue or its source.

Here are some stress-relief methods that I share with people to help them put their bodies into a more relaxed state:

- ✓ Freeze your face. This is an odd technique I learned a long time ago. During the course of your day, stop what you are doing, and "freeze" your face. Bring your attention to your expression. Notice if the eyebrows are furrowed, if the jaw is clenched, and whether you are smiling or not. When you freeze your face, you capture a snapshot that might reveal some interesting things to you. As always, you want to observe without judging. When you are informed, it can help you to make a conscious decision to be aware of what is displayed to the world. I used to be always in thinking mode until one day someone asked me why I looked so mad all the time. Here I was simply thinking, thinking, thinking, and I was appearing angry to the outside world. I pondered this more and remembered the freeze your face technique that I had learned as a child. It is now part of my daily check-in, and I'm happy to say that I'm more conscious about sharing joy with the outer world. Consciously relax your jaw muscles, and unfurrow your brow. Let yourself *smile*.

✓ Hold a rock. Find a stone that has the specific purpose of helping you relax. Many crystals and stones are suited to helping you feel calmer. Everything is energy, so find a stone that suits your needs and responds to your vibration. Lepidolite, howlite, and aventurine are a few suggestions.

✓ Take a walk. Reconnect with the earth. Get out, get fresh air, and feel grounded. Take three deep breaths to fill your lungs. Being out in nature can rejuvenate your soul! Get outside at least once a day, no matter the weather, and allow yourself to fully see the colors, see the trees, and feel the earth below your feet. Bring awareness to the beauty and connection of all.

✓ Shake it up. Bounce up and down, shake, rattle, and move your body. Your muscles are begging to be used. When you bounce or shake, you release any stuck energy. Dance, walk, stretch, and connect with yourself through body awareness.

✓ Use your phone. Put your phone to good use! Here is a tip I find extremely helpful. Program your phone to go off every few hours with a reminder to take a deep breath. Sometimes I get the reminder at the most convenient times. This is a great way to use the phone to help you relax.

✓ Say it again. Mantras and affirmations really do work! Repetition is the key. When you keep repeating a positive word or a phrase, say it like you mean it. This will help program your subconscious mind. Words are powerful, so allow the energy of each word you recite to uplift you and take you to a place deep within your heart. Say the following words softly to yourself as you focus on the energy:

- Nurture
- Relax
- Sustain
- Harmony

- Oneness
- Soften
- Serenity
- Peacefulness
- Bliss
- Calm
- Hope
- Balance
- Flow
- Joy
- Embrace
- Warmth
- Surrender
- Divine
- Love

✓ Practice before you need it. It's easier to develop a practice in times of grace and ease. Set aside time each day to sit and reflect. Honor yourself, and take a moment to appreciate how far you've come.

Learning to incorporate mindfulness into your everyday life will help provide you with the tools to relieve stress. Let go of things you cannot control, take a deep breath, and *relax*.

Day Twenty-One

Trust yourself. Create the kind of self that you will be happy to live with all your life. Make the most of yourself by fanning the tiny, inner sparks of possibility into flames of achievement.

—Golda Meir

Affirmation

"I celebrate my progress and will continue to grow."

Crystal

Today's crystal is hematite.

Focus

Congratulate yourself on completing this Divine Dining Method program! Hopefully you feel as though your relationship with food has become more mindful through the practice of meditation and self-reflection. If you continue to need a helping hand, return to either the seven-day workbook or this twenty-one-day guide to help you in the practice of the Divine Dining Method! Thank you for letting me share this journey with you.

Journal

Record your meals and any thoughts that came to you during your morning meditation. Take a few minutes to reflect on your journey. What changes have you noticed in the way you think about food and the way you interact with it? What about your self-esteem and confidence levels? What do you still hope to accomplish?

Recommended Reading: Your Only Job

Our only job is to be an example of a life that is working.

—Marianne Williamson

The above quote touches me deeply. The more we look into our own lives as they are in this moment, the more we are able to make the changes necessary. My coaching training has taught me to look at my life from all angles and come into acceptance for all. When you examine all aspects of your life, you can see where things are not working as well what is working. This is all about telling the raw truth to yourself, which is the key to moving forward. Said differently, it is when we accept where we are in this moment that we can move toward that which we desire.

Have you ever had the luxury of completely dwelling in your heart? If so, how did it feel? When you are conscious of your inner world you live more fully within the rhythm of your heart. How can you continue to excavate your inner world to find more of the gold within? We know that anything that is not of the light will be brought up to the surface for us to look at and examine. Then it is up to us to own it and release it. These are the steps to freedom.

How can you dig more deeply into the treasures of your heart? What is the thread you use to weave the fabric of your life? Is it made of trust and faith, together with optimism and gratitude? And is this thread created from the golden strands from the depths of your soul? Seeing this as opportunity to stitch a new foundation, what is it that you want most in this time? Do you want a sense of peace to cover you like a blanket?

After all that we have been through, isn't it nice to know that we can depend on ourselves? Not to overstate things, but it is our inner landscape that means the most. What is your inner world like in this moment? Are you filled with trust and peace? Are you weeding away remnants of discontent?

It is when we disengage from the outer drama that we can find a true sense of peace. Our thoughts can run amok, and we can get swept up in the frenzy. Choose to honor your heart, and choose to dwell there more often. Clean up your inner world. Get to the cobwebs in the corners of your soul. Do the excavation. As you do, your consciousness expands. Be grateful for all the treasures in your heart. Surround yourself with all that uplifts and expands you. Get back to your groove, and feel the rhythm of your soul. Enjoy the job of your life—and may you find contentment and courage to move ahead.

AFTERWORD

Thank you so much for joining me on this journey into the Divine Dining Method. I hope you'll return to this book over and over again.

Remember, the journey isn't over; it is just beginning!

I leave you with this: if I were to simplify the Divine Dining Method, I would tell you to try these three tips:

- ✓ *Focus* on the food you eat while you are eating.
- ✓ *Pause* to take a deep breath before your first bite.
- ✓ *Appreciate* and be *grateful* for your food (where it came from and who prepared it).

REFERENCES

Albers, Susan. *Eat, Drink, and Be Mindful.* Oakland, California: New Harbinger Publications, 2008

Altman, Donald. *Meal by Meal: 365 Daily Meditations for Finding Balance through Mindful Eating.* Novato, California: New World Library 2004

Epstein, Catherine Russo. *Divine Dining, Sea Cliff New York; 2006.*

Epstein, Catherine Russo. *Gateways of Inspiration.* Sea Cliff, New York: Lulu Publishing, 2008

Hanh, Thich Nhat. *How to Eat.* Berkeley, California: Parallax Press 2014

Kabat-Zinn, Jon. *Letting Everything Be Your Teacher: 100 Lessons in Mindfulness.* New York, New York: Bantam Bell, 2009

Nepo, Mark. *The Book of Awakening: Having the Life You Want by Being Present to the Life You Have.* San Fransisco, California: Conari Press 2000